Rethinking Rural Governance
Volume 1 — Delaware County, New York
From Compliance to Systems Intelligence

Published under the SozoRock Foundation Modernization and Resilience Program

Printed in the United States of America

© 2025 The SozoRock Foundation, New York. All rights reserved.
No portion of this publication may be reproduced, stored, or transmitted in any form or by any means—electronic, mechanical, photocopying, recording, or otherwise—without prior written permission from The SozoRock Foundation. Brief excerpts may be quoted for academic, journalistic, or policy analysis when properly cited.

ISBN 979-8-9936477-1-5
Published and distributed by The SozoRock Foundation • New York

Preferred citation
Adeyemo, O. (2025). *Rethinking Rural Governance: Volume 1 – Delaware County, New York — From Compliance to Systems Intelligence.* The SozoRock Foundation, New York.

Editorial Office. Modernization and Resilience Program
www.sozorockfoundation.org
contact@sozorockfoundation.org

Sustainable governance begins when compliance evolves into continuous learning.

Series Intent

The Rethinking Rural Governance series examines how counties and provinces can convert administrative compliance into systems intelligence. It studies how fiscal design, workforce discipline, and data architecture combine to strengthen the capacity of small and mid-scale governments to plan, decide, and adapt.

Each volume translates verified public data into operational frameworks that link efficiency with equity—building models of governance that learn continuously and earn trust over time.

Series Overview

Rural jurisdictions across North America face similar pressures: aging populations, workforce shortages, and limited data integration. The Rethinking Rural Governance series addresses these conditions through evidence and design.

It documents practical mechanisms that enable counties and provincial systems to sustain essential services, strengthen accountability, and modernize institutional performance without urban scale.

Developed under The SozoRock Foundation's Modernization and Resilience Program, the series supports replication of effective modernization strategies across U.S. and Canadian contexts—advancing governance as a system of foresight, transparency, and national resilience.

National and Binational Modernization Value

County modernization needs across the United States increasingly reflect a shared structural pattern: aging populations, workforce shortages, fiscal complexity, and rising compliance demands. Similar pressures appear in rural regions across the Midwest, the Mountain West, and in Ontario and British Columbia, where local governments manage expanding responsibilities with limited administrative capacity. These converging trends create an environment where counties must meet higher expectations with tools and systems designed for an earlier decade.

This alignment presents a shared opportunity. The modernization model introduced in this volume—systems intelligence, capability sequencing, and evidence-based governance—operates as a transferable framework for jurisdictions working with constrained workforces, growing mandates, and static fiscal flexibility. The principles outlined here describe the institutional architecture required to support modernization while maintaining continuity of essential services.

The methodology reflects an emerging standard for practical, capability-based administrative reform.

Three attributes position this framework for national and binational impact

Scalable architecture

The model applies to counties and municipalities of varying sizes and structures. Its strength lies in focusing on capabilities rather than organizational scale, enabling adoption by jurisdictions with either limited staff or broad departmental networks.

Cross-system integration

Aligning public health, fiscal management, compliance operations, and community literacy within a single modernization sequence reduces the fragmentation that shapes decision-making across North American regions.

Forward-looking governance

The emphasis on intelligence, learning, and operational foresight strengthens readiness for future public-health requirements, fiscal shifts, and administrative challenges. This aligns with federal modernization priorities and with modernization agendas within Canadian provincial systems.

As more regions explore practical pathways to modernization, the approach documented in this volume demonstrates how counties can move from reactive administration to systems-oriented governance. It provides a shared structure for leaders working to strengthen resilience, improve institutional performance, and support long-term preparedness in both the United States and Canada. Widespread adoption of this capability model can contribute to a more coherent modernization agenda—building public systems that allocate resources more effectively and sustain long-term resilience across North America.

At a Glance

Indicator & Insight

$4.8 million
Total 2024 public health expenditure — fiscal stability with categorical-aid dependency.

58%
Proportion of expenditures financed by state and federal grants, limiting fiscal flexibility.

27%
Residents aged 60+ — the fastest-growing population segment.

12%
County poverty rate — a key driver of health and mobility needs.

13%
Households experiencing food insecurity.

3 Modernization Levers
- Fiscal Intelligence
- Workforce Analytics
- Community Transparency

Target Horizon 2028
County projected to achieve adaptive systems intelligence within four fiscal cycles.

Summary

Delaware County exemplifies the transition from stable compliance to emergent systems intelligence. Verified fiscal discipline, workforce investments, and data transparency now position the county as a replicable model for rural modernization in both the United States and Canada.

Foreword

Rural governance is entering a new era. The challenge is no longer one of accountability alone, but of agility—the ability to anticipate rather than react. For counties balancing aging demographics, static revenues, and expanding service demands, modernization is not optional; it is the foundation of long-term resilience.

The Rethinking Rural Governance series provides an analytical pathway for that transformation.

Delaware County, New York, serves as the inaugural case because of its verified transparency, disciplined fiscal management, and measurable progress toward systems intelligence.

The SozoRock Foundation created this series to document, not idealize, the work of rural administrators who are redefining what responsible governance looks like in the twenty-first century. This first volume demonstrates that modernization is achievable wherever evidence, discipline, and vision intersect.

Oluwabiyi Adeyemo

Director, Strategic Initiatives

The SozoRock Foundation

Table of Contents

At a Glance
Foreword
Executive Summary

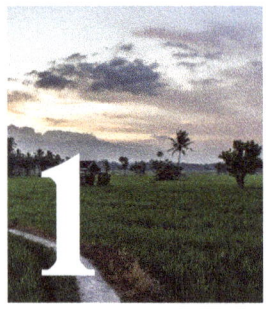 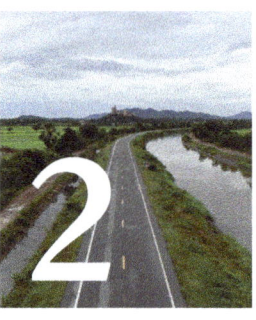 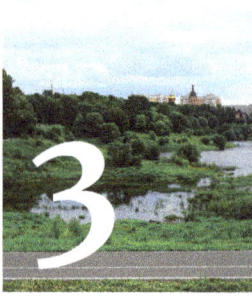 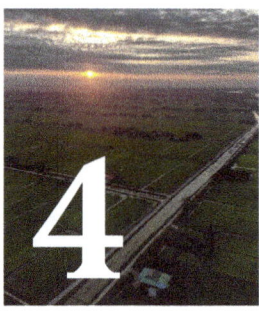 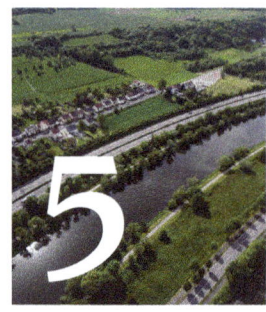

Governance and Modernization Context	Findings from Verified County Data — Analytical Core	Systems Intelligence Framework for Rural Governance	Strategic Outlook and Scalability Potential	Appendices and Data References
Defining Systems Intelligence	Funding and Fiscal Intelligence	Framework Structure	National Relevance and Policy Alignment	Documentary Sources and Verification
Fiscal Discipline and Structural Constraints	Workforce Modernization	Core Components of the Framework	Strategic Pathways for U.S. Replication	Analytical Methodology
Workforce Readiness and Continuity	Chronic Disease and Preventive Health Trends	Operational Model — From Compliance to Intelligence	Cross-Border Application — Ontario and Beyond	Framework Definitions and Terminology
Community Determinants and Data Integration	Maternal and Child Health Programs	Systems Design for Rural Replication	Funding and Sustainability Mechanisms	Acknowledgments
Comparative Perspective	Environmental Health and Safety Systems	Governance Intelligence Metrics	Institutional Scalability Model	Replication and Licensing Notice
Cross-Border Scalability	Emergency Preparedness and Institutional Resilience	Strategic Path Forward	National Impact and Future Outlook	Series Continuation Plan
	Integrated Systems Perspective	Cross-Border Scalability	Concluding Outlook	Citation and Contact
	Modernization Trajectory	Summary Insight		End Note

Executive Summary

$4.8 million
Total 2024–2025 public-health expenditures in Delaware County.

$2.8 million
Covered by state and federal aid.

$2 million
Approximate net county cost after external aid.

Delaware County, New York, exemplifies both the achievements and the constraints of a maturing rural governance model. Fiscal discipline and transparent operations are evident in verified 2024–2025 reports, with total public-health expenditures near $4.8 million and $2.8 million covered by state and federal aid—leaving roughly $2 million in net county cost. The fiscal composition illustrates a structural reality for many rural counties: predictable revenue, constrained flexibility, and limited data capacity for real-time resource alignment.

Insight

Financial control is solid, but flexibility remains constrained by categorical aid and limited real-time analytics.

Figure 1
Fiscal Composition, Delaware County 2024

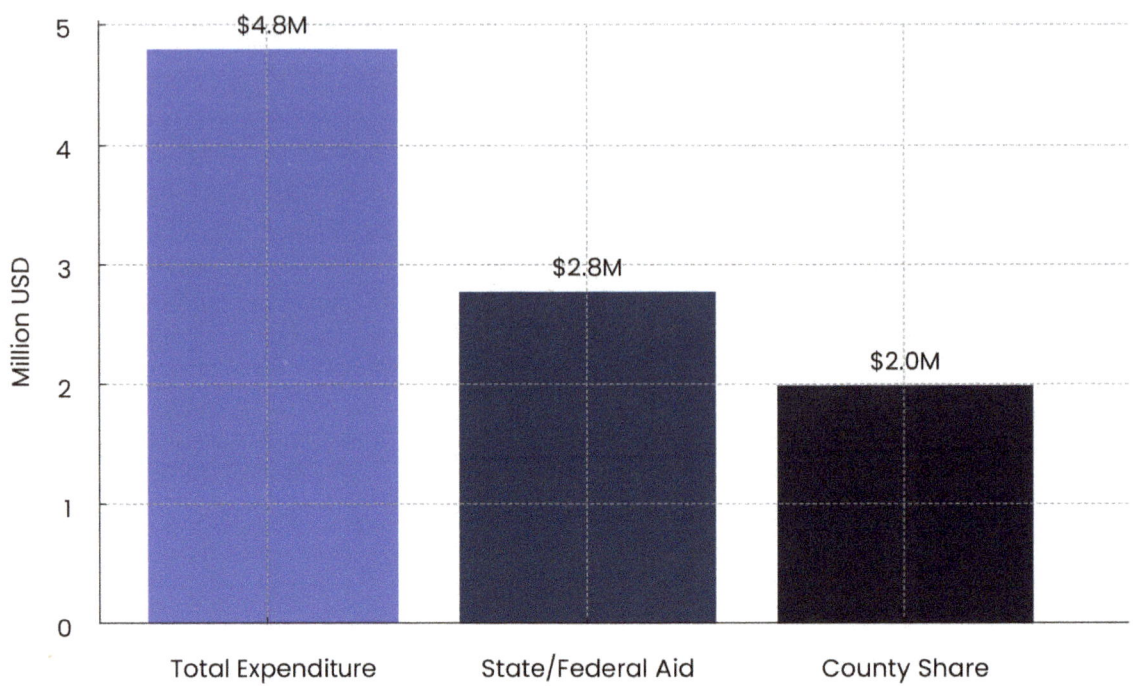

Source: Delaware County Public Health Services (2024 Annual Report); SozoRock Foundation analysis.

Insight

Public-health funding remains stable yet structurally dependent on categorical aid. Roughly 58 percent of expenditures rely on external sources, limiting fiscal agility and innovation.

Operationally, approximately 12 percent of the health budget was dedicated to workforce stabilization through the Public Health Infrastructure Grant. The investment improved retention and morale, supported digital upgrades, and ensured continuity of essential services. Structurally, the county still lacks integrated analytics to link staffing trends with projected service demand—a gap that limits long-term workforce intelligence.

Insight

Workforce resilience has strengthened, but without integrated forecasting, long-term intelligence remains out of reach.

Programmatically, the 2024 Annual Report underscores strength across communicable-disease control, lead prevention, maternal-child health, emergency preparedness, and chronic-disease education. Each fulfills state compliance standards yet functions as a discrete vertical. The modernization challenge is to integrate these data streams under a shared systems-intelligence framework capable of turning operational reporting into predictive insight.

Compliance is achieved, but integration is the next frontier.

Demographically, the county faces an aging population—over 27 percent aged 60 or older—combined with rising food insecurity (13 percent of households) and mobility limitations (8 percent lacking private transportation). Poverty affects roughly 12 percent of residents, with disproportionate impact on single-parent and elderly households. These factors collectively pressure service delivery and justify an analytical shift from procedural reporting toward predictive planning.

Aging, mobility, and economic vulnerability create persistent service strain, reinforcing the need for predictive planning.

Figure 2
Demographic Pressures: Aging vs Poverty (2015-2024)

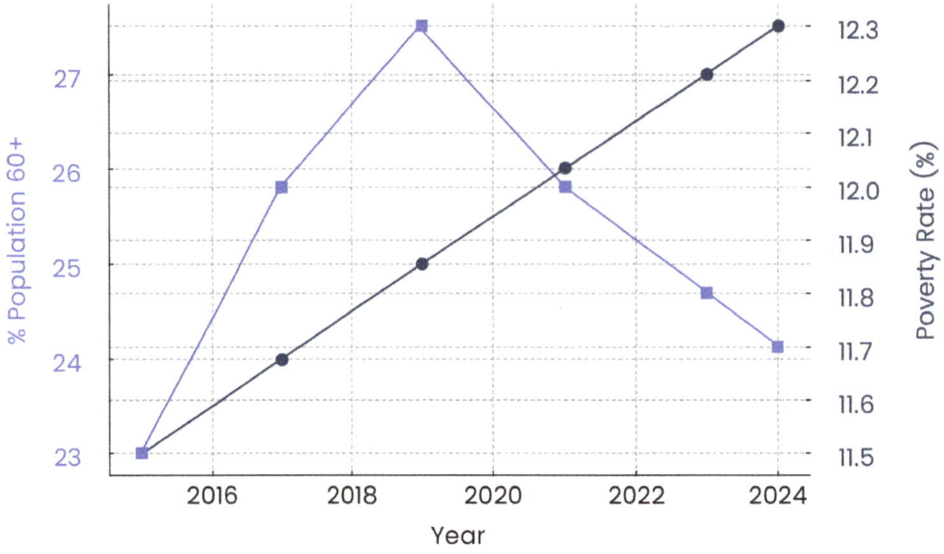

Source: Delaware County Community Health Assessment (2022-2024); SozoRock Foundation analysis.

Insight

Delaware County faces a converging demographic strain. The share of residents aged 60+ has risen steadily over the past decade, while poverty levels remain persistently near 12 percent. This dual trend increases pressure on workforce capacity, transport systems, and county fiscal stability—intensifying the need for integrated planning and modernization.

To manage these structural shifts, three capability levers are essential:

1. **Institutional Systems Intelligence** – Enable multi-program integration so aging-population trends, poverty indicators, and service utilization patterns inform forecasting, resourcing, and operational decisions.
2. **Workforce and Governance Modernization** – Strengthen county workforce pipelines, digital skills, and administrative processes to support rising demand for aging services and cross-agency coordination.
3. **Community Literacy and Transparency** – Expand evidence-informed communication, digital literacy, and public-facing data tools so community partners and residents can engage more effectively in planning and compliance requirements.

These pressures highlight why governance modernization—and the ability to convert dispersed county data into actionable intelligence—has become essential.

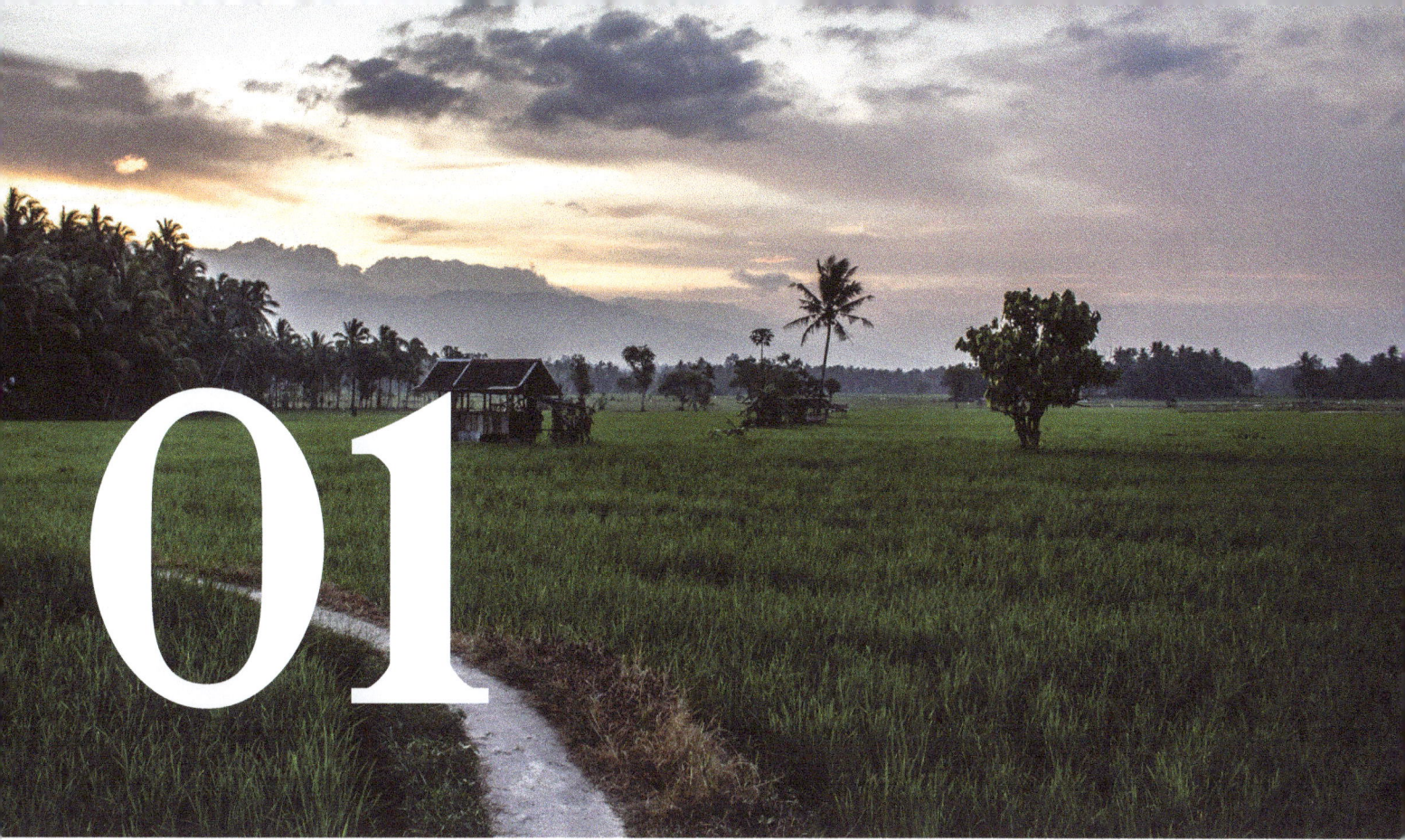

01

Governance and Modernization Context

Administratively, Delaware County demonstrates continuity and accountability through its Health Services Advisory Board and associated program networks. Verified 2025 minutes record disciplined fiscal oversight, structured grant acceptance, and transparent reporting—foundations of sound governance. Yet these same records reveal latent opportunity: extensive data capture without systematic translation into strategic intelligence.

Defining Systems Intelligence

Systems intelligence denotes the capacity of a county administration to translate dispersed financial, workforce, and program data into a consolidated analytics environment that anticipates needs, aligns resources, and measures performance in real time. Establishing this capability is the cornerstone of modern rural governance.

Fiscal Discipline and Structural Constraints

The 2024 Public Health Services Annual Report demonstrates fiscal steadiness yet dependence on categorical grants that limit flexibility. Modernization requires embedding analytics within budgeting cycles so departments can forecast service loads rather than merely reconcile expenses.

Workforce Readiness

Minutes from early 2025 confirm ongoing recruitment of nurses, coordinators, and therapists—evidence of proactive leadership. However, absence of longitudinal analytics prevents visibility into retention trends, tenure patterns, or skill alignment. Embedding workforce dashboards would elevate staffing from transactional management to predictive capacity design.

Community Determinants and Data Integration

The 2022–2024 Community Health Assessment identifies transportation, income disparity, housing stability, and food insecurity as persistent determinants. Without integrated dashboards linking these indicators to outcomes, insight remains static. A unified data platform—supported by standardized governance—would enable visualization of system performance and resource efficiency.

Comparative Perspective

Delaware County's modernization posture aligns with peer counties adopting performance-based frameworks since 2022: strong compliance infrastructure, emerging digital capacity, and limited cross-system analytics. Its readiness to institutionalize intelligence places it at an inflection point for national learning.

Cross-Border Scalability

Comparable demographic and administrative conditions in rural Ontario mirror Delaware's modernization landscape. Frameworks emerging here could inform bilateral collaboration under SozoRock's broader systems-resilience initiative, positioning rural governance as a shared North American modernization frontier.

Operationally, the county's engagement with DataGen Inc. to extend the assessment framework through 2030 demonstrates forward intent. Structurally, embedding that framework into a countywide intelligence architecture would ensure every report contributes to real-time analytics. Strategically, such integration converts compliance data into foresight—transforming Delaware County from a well-managed jurisdiction into a continuously learning system.

The next section interprets verified county data across six domains—funding, workforce, chronic-disease trends, environmental health, maternal-child outcomes, and emergency preparedness—to identify measurable modernization levers.

Figure 3
Governance Intelligence Maturity Map

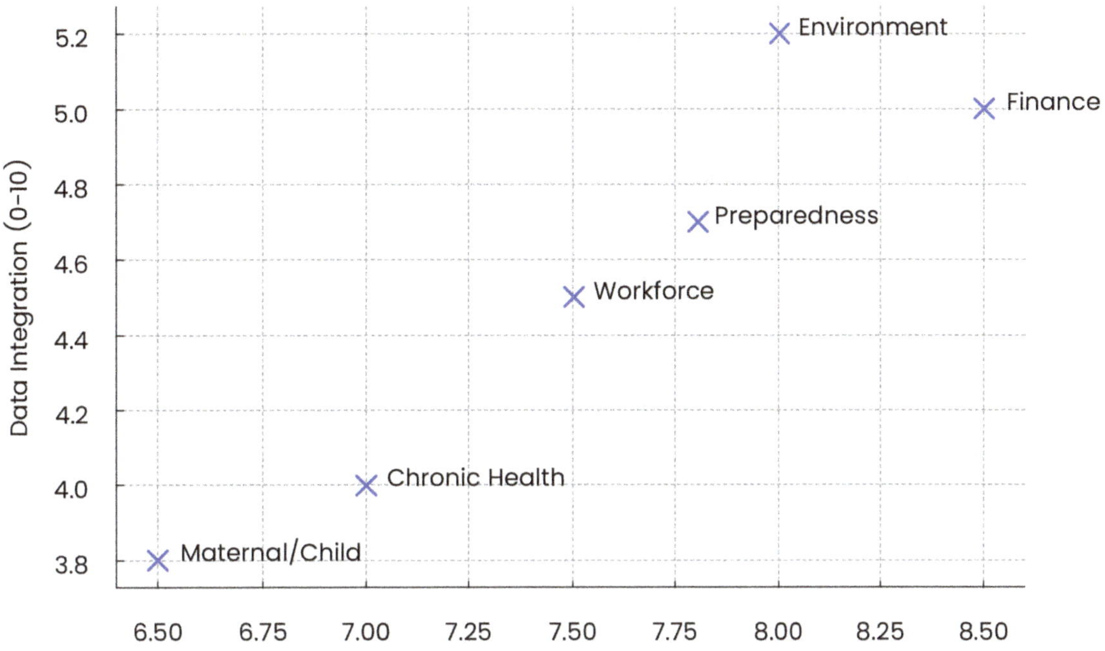

[Scatter plot with Data Integration (0-10) on y-axis ranging from 3.8 to 5.2, and x-axis ranging from 6.50 to 8.50. Points plotted:
- Environment: (~8.0, 5.2)
- Finance: (~8.5, 5.0)
- Preparedness: (~7.8, 4.7)
- Workforce: (~7.5, 4.5)
- Chronic Health: (~7.0, 4.0)
- Maternal/Child: (~6.5, 3.8)]

Source: Delaware County Public Health Services (2024–2025) and SozoRock Foundation analysis.

Performance across six county domains reveals a consistent pattern: strong execution strength paired with limited data integration. Delaware County delivers reliably in core operations—particularly in environment, finance, and preparedness—yet lacks unified data structures, reducing visibility intro trends, outcomes, and cross-system interactions. Maternal/Child Health and Chronic Health remain the least integrated domains, highlighting priority areas for modernization.

Insight

Delaware County demonstrates high operational strength but fragmented intelligence. Most domains perform well day-to-day, yet their data systems operate in silos, limiting forecasting, risk detection, and coordinated planning. The largest modernization gains will come from elevating low-integration domains—Maternal/Child Health and Chronic Health—and extending shared analytics across Environment, Finance, Workforce, and Preparedness.

Governance Intelligence Maturity Pathway

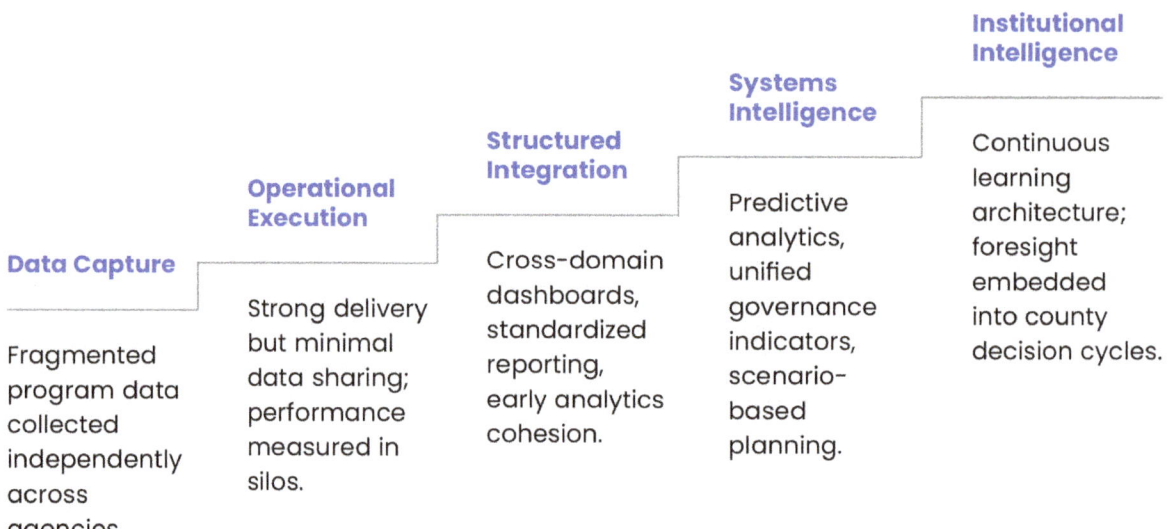

Data Capture
Fragmented program data collected independently across agencies.

Operational Execution
Strong delivery but minimal data sharing; performance measured in silos.

Structured Integration
Cross-domain dashboards, standardized reporting, early analytics cohesion.

Systems Intelligence
Predictive analytics, unified governance indicators, scenario-based planning.

Institutional Intelligence
Continuous learning architecture; foresight embedded into county decision cycles.

County modernization advances as data moves from fragmented capture to institutional intelligence—keeping execution strong while elevating strategic capability.

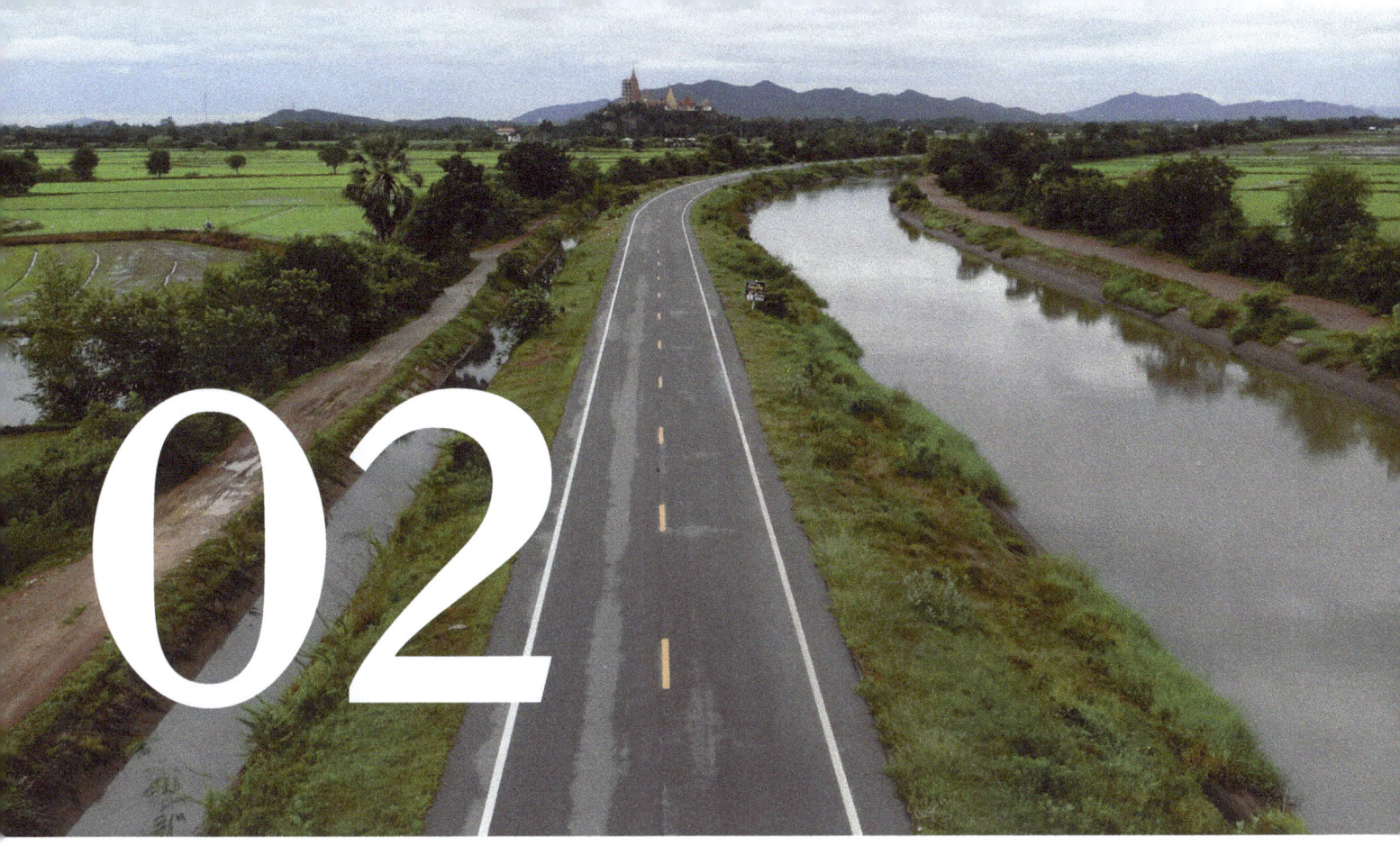

02

Findings from Verified County Data — Analytical Core

Delaware County's verified public records for 2024–2025 reveal a governance system that is fiscally disciplined yet structurally constrained. The Health Services Advisory Board minutes, the Public Health Services Annual Report, and the 2022–2024 Community Health Assessment (CHA) collectively map a county transitioning from program delivery to organizational modernization. Each dataset exposes one consistent pattern — strong execution, limited integration.

$4.8 million
Total Public Health expenditures in 2024.

$2.8 million
State and federal aid received.

$2 million
Locally funded through property-tax allocations and revenue transfers.

Funding and Fiscal Intelligence

Findings

County records confirm total Public Health expenditures reached ≈ $4.8 million in 2024, with $2.8 million in state and federal aid. The balance—slightly above $2 million—was borne locally through property-tax allocations and revenue transfers. Roughly one-third of this budget is locked into mandated programs, reducing flexibility for innovation. The pattern illustrates a predictable but rigid structure: categorical grants sustain continuity while masking efficiency opportunities.

Minutes from the March 2025 session note routine acceptance of Article 6 contracts but no discussion of fiscal dashboards or predictive tools. Reconciliation remains a quarterly obligation rather than a planning exercise. The absence of an interactive financial architecture prevents scenario testing or impact projection.

Modernization Lever Insight

Develop a county-wide fiscal-intelligence module synthesizing program costs, grant cycles, and staffing allocations into a single analytics view. Such a platform shifts budgeting from compliance to foresight.

Workforce Modernization

Findings

Workforce stability dominated 2024–2025. Minutes from January and June 2025 confirm multiple recruitments for nursing and environmental staff, financed by the Public Health Infrastructure Grant. Workspace upgrades and wellness initiatives improved morale and retention amid statewide shortages.

Yet no comprehensive workforce-analytics system tracks turnover, training, or competency alignment. Data reside in program files, not an integrated human-capital dashboard. Personnel reports are reviewed for cost compliance, not predictive capacity.

Modernization Lever Insight

Institutionalize workforce intelligence by linking HR records to program and service-volume data. This enables forecasting, succession planning, and measurable returns on training investments.

≥ 25 percent

Population aged 60+ in Delaware County, indicating an aging demographic and higher chronic disease risk.

Chronic Disease and Preventive Health Trends

Findings

The CHA identifies chronic illness—diabetes, hypertension, obesity—as Delaware County's leading health burden. An aging population (≥ 25 percent aged 60 +) and limited transportation amplify risk. Preventive programming remains educational rather than data-driven; metrics track event attendance, not behavioral change or screening outcomes.

Modernization Lever Insight

Create a chronic-disease intelligence dashboard linking hospital discharges, screenings, and demographics to target resources in real time and model population risk.

Maternal and Child Health Programs

Findings

The Maternal and Child Health Program maintains home visits, immunization clinics, and lead screening with steady participation. Manual recordkeeping, however, limits evaluation; updates in minutes list cases, not developmental outcomes.

Modernization Lever Insight

Adopt a digital maternal-child registry integrated with public-health databases for longitudinal tracking of risk factors and outcomes—turning compliance data into evidence for policy design.

Environmental Health and Safety Systems

Findings

Annual reports document robust inspection activity in water, septic, and food-service oversight. Despite staff turnover, performance remained steady through manual workflows. Paper forms and spreadsheets dominate; real-time reporting is absent.

Modernization Lever Insight

Deploy a geospatial environmental-health system connecting inspection data to GIS layers for faster risk detection, trend analysis, and transparent public updates.

Emergency Preparedness and Institutional Resilience

Findings

Emergency Preparedness appears consistently in 2024–2025 records. Plans for outbreak response and mass dispensing are updated and tested through drills, yet after-action results stay narrative and unquantified. Integration with data systems remains partial.

> **Modernization Lever Insight**
>
> Implement a Resilience Operations Dashboard aggregating alerts, hospital capacity, and supply inventories for simulation, coordination, and real-time crisis response.

Integrated Systems Perspective

Across all domains, the dominant theme is fragmentation. Delaware County maintains rich documentation but lacks interoperability. Governance maturity is evident; intelligence maturity is emerging.

The transition requires a unifying architecture where every dataset reinforces strategic foresight.

Modernization Trajectory

Building on verified data, Delaware County is positioned to pioneer a rural systems-intelligence framework grounded in three structural transformations:

- **From Records to Intelligence —** Consolidate datasets across finance, workforce, and health programs to enable unified analytics.
- **From Reactive to Predictive Governance —** Embed analytics into budgeting and evaluation cycles.
- **From Compliance to Continuous Learning —** Establish feedback loops where outcomes inform future planning.

When fully integrated, these transformations elevate Delaware County from a compliant jurisdiction to a model of rural governance intelligence—a blueprint adaptable nationwide and across Ontario's rural regions.

Source: Delaware County verified budget records (2024–2025) and SozoRock Foundation projection.

Insight

Modernization advances when counties treat data systems as living infrastructure-stabilizing records, integrating intelligence, and embedding continuous learning into governance cycles.

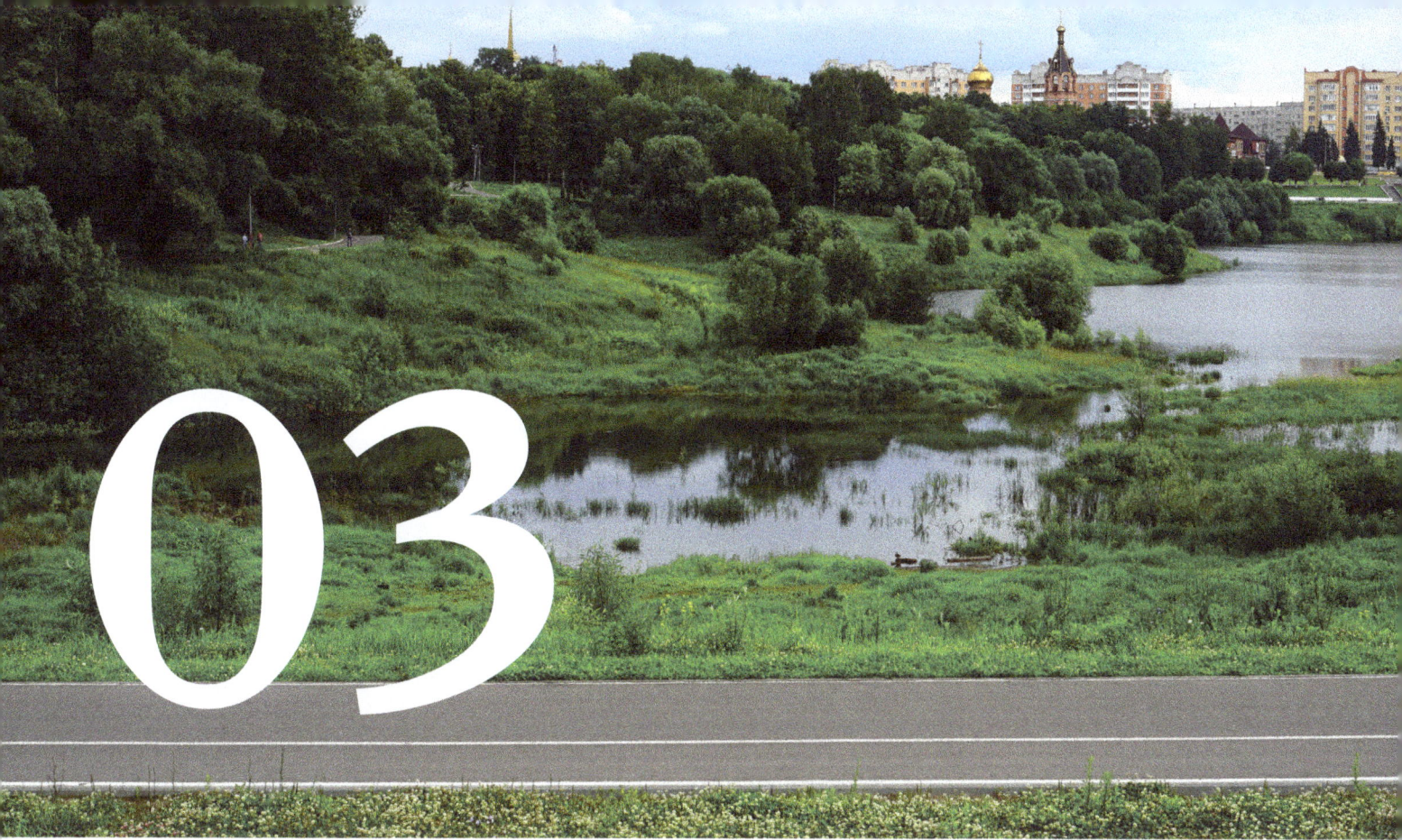

03

Systems Intelligence Framework for Rural Governance

Delaware County's modernization trajectory defines a scalable model for converting rural administrative systems from procedural compliance to adaptive intelligence.

This framework—derived from verified county data and SozoRock's modernization benchmarks—translates the evidence base into an operational discipline rather than a conceptual ambition.

Figure 4
Three-Tier Systems Intelligence Model

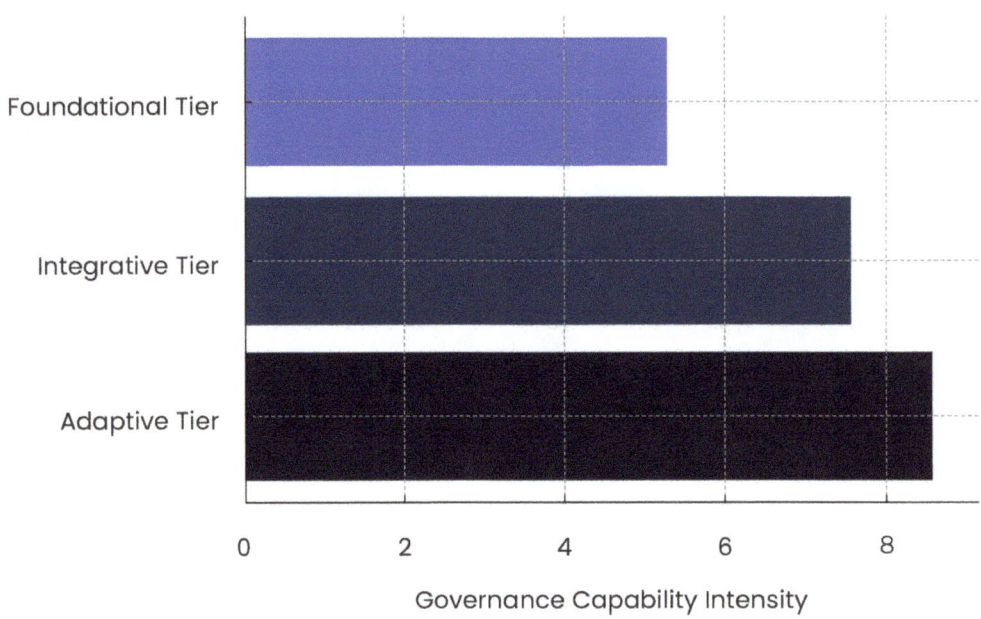

Source: SozoRock Foundation Systems Resilience Framework (2025).

Governance capability evolves in three maturity layers, moving from data visibility toward learning-based intelligence.

Insight

Delaware County demonstrates high execution strength but low data integration—revealing strong operations but fragmented intelligence.

Framework Structure

Systems intelligence develops through three tiers of maturity, each representing a distinct capability layer within governance operations.

1. Foundational Tier — Data Integrity and Visibility

Reliable capture of fiscal, workforce, and program data is the starting point. Delaware County's current records meet compliance requirements but lack shared visibility. Establishing unified data standards, validated storage, and cross-department dashboards will convert static reports into real-time administrative assets.

2. Integrative Tier — Analytics and Decision Linkages

Once visibility exists, analytics must interconnect finance, workforce, and community outcomes. Predictive tools—budget forecasting, attrition modeling, and risk profiling—enable leaders to anticipate rather than react. Fiscal and health metrics merged in a single platform yield foresight instead of after-action review.

3. Adaptive Tier — Continuous Learning and Governance Foresight

At full maturity, systems intelligence institutionalizes learning. Departments exchange insights automatically; reports generate metrics; leadership decisions trigger feedback loops that refine policy. Governance becomes a self-updating system of knowledge.

Core Components of the Framework

1. Governance Data Architecture

County documentation is thorough yet dispersed. Creating a central data warehouse integrating fiscal ledgers, workforce files, and CHA/CHIP indicators forms the structural backbone of systems intelligence. Data-access protocols and validation audits ensure integrity and confidentiality.

2. Performance Analytics Engine

The analytical layer transforms records into dashboards. For Delaware County, quarterly Board data can be modeled to link cost centers with outcome indicators—producing actionable performance insights.

3. Feedback and Learning Loop

Board reviews are currently qualitative. Embedding automated feedback loops—surveys, dashboards, and time-series visualizations—turns every decision into measurable evidence for improvement.

4. Workforce Capability System

Recruitment and retention reports show stability but no analytics on skill deployment. Integrating HR data with program outcomes establishes a dynamic workforce-planning tool tied to service demand.

5. Community Transparency Interface

Open dashboards for fiscal, environmental, and health metrics reinforce accountability. Public access to verified summaries transforms governance intelligence into civic literacy.

Operational Model — From Compliance to Intelligence

Phase	Operational Focus	Deliverables	Governance Outcome
Phase I – Data Stabilization (Years 1–2)	Standardize capture, validate reports	Unified templates, baseline dashboards	Reliable information environment
Phase II – Integration and Analytics (Years 2–3)	Cross-domain data links, predictive tools	Workforce & fiscal modeling dashboards	Early decision intelligence
Phase III – Learning Governance (Year 4 +)	Feedback loops, community dashboards	Annual modernization index	Fully adaptive governance system

Progress is measured through quantifiable indicators—number of datasets integrated, frequency of data-driven decisions, and audit-response efficiency.

Figure 5
Operational Phasing Roadmap (Years 1–4+)

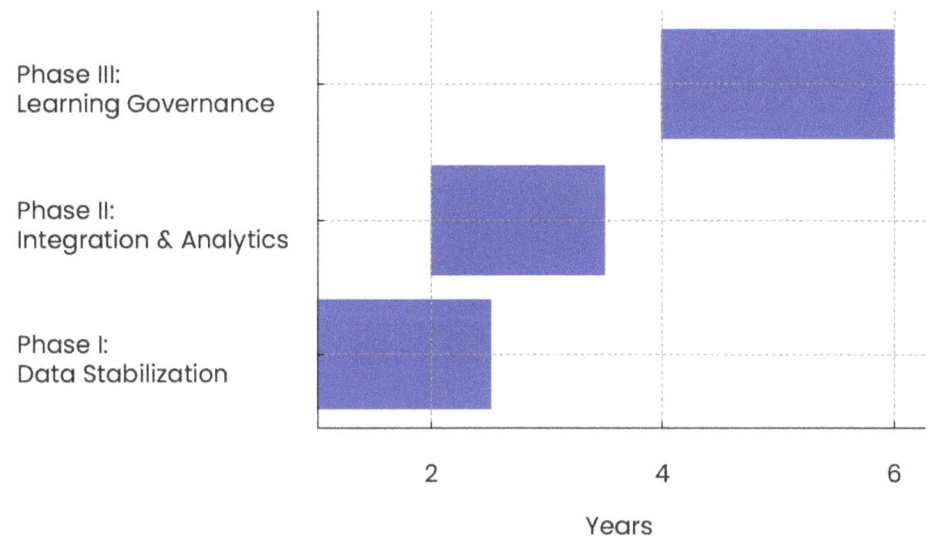

Source Note: Delaware County verified records (2024–2025); SozoRock Foundation projection (2025).

Delaware County's modernization journey follows a four-year phasing model— data stabilization, integration, and adaptive governance.

Systems Design for Rural Replication

The Delaware County framework can scale across rural counties and comparable Ontario regions where administrative scale and demographics align.

- **Interoperability Standard:** Adopt open-data protocols compatible with state and provincial systems.
- **Governance Consortium:** Form inter-county exchanges to share dashboards and metrics annually.
- **Capacity Partnerships:** Engage universities and colleges to co-deliver analytics and digital-literacy training.
- **Public Engagement Layer:** Extend dashboards to libraries and community hubs to promote rural data literacy.

Together these mechanisms establish a Rural Governance Modernization Network linking U.S. and Canadian jurisdictions through shared intelligence standards.

Governance Intelligence Metrics

Category	Indicator	Purpose
Fiscal Intelligence	Ratio of predictive to retrospective budget actions	Measure shift to proactive planning
Workforce Analytics	% of positions linked to dashboards	Gauge penetration of intelligence systems
Program Integration	Number of cross-department datasets	Quantify interoperability
Learning Loop Adoption	Frequency of post-decision data reviews	Assess continuous learning culture
Transparency Index	Quarterly public dashboard updates	Track open-governance progress

These metrics convert modernization from concept to accountability.

Strategic Path Forward

To institutionalize systems intelligence, Delaware County should:

- Finalize a Data Governance Charter defining ownership and interoperability.
- Establish a Modernization Team uniting department leads and analytics staff.
- Launch a Fiscal & Workforce Dashboard Pilot as proof of value.
- Develop a Modernization Index benchmarking annual progress against peer counties.

Such measures bridge the current compliance structure with the adaptive intelligence required for long-term resilience.

Cross-Border Scalability

Ontario's rural counties face similar demographic and infrastructural dynamics. Aligning Delaware's framework with provincial modernization agendas enables binational cooperation under SozoRock's Systems Resilience Program. Shared definitions, training modules, and metrics will create an interoperable North-American rural-governance standard.

Summary Insight

Systems intelligence is less a technology than a discipline—treating data as infrastructure, decisions as experiments, and feedback as governance capital. Through this disciplined approach, Delaware County—and by extension, rural America—can evolve into institutions that learn continuously, anticipate needs, and sustain national resilience.

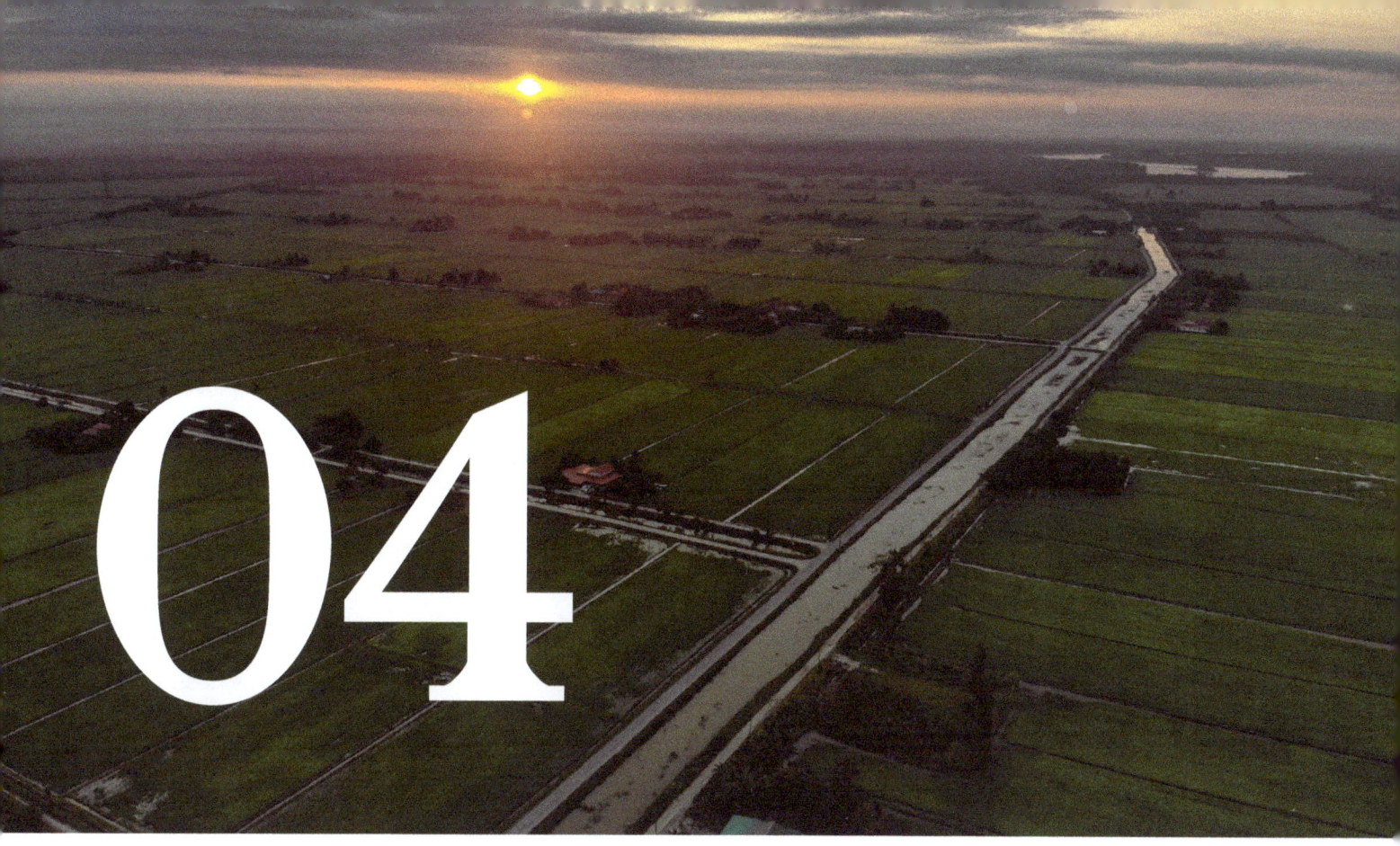

04

Strategic Outlook and Scalability Potential

Delaware County's modernization work demonstrates how a rural jurisdiction can move from reactive compliance toward a self-learning governance system with national relevance.

The county's experience establishes an operational precedent for replication across the United States and comparable regions of Canada, where similar demographic and fiscal constraints prevail.

National Relevance and Policy Alignment

Modernization within Delaware County aligns with both state and federal modernization agendas.

At the U.S. level, the Department of Health and Human Services' Data Modernization Initiative and the CDC's local data-capacity goals emphasize real-time intelligence for health and resilience.

At the state level, New York's Prevention Agenda 2025–2030 mandates cross-sector data integration and equity metrics for every county.

The systems-intelligence framework implemented through SozoRock's methodology directly supports these goals. Its fiscal-intelligence layer advances transparency and resource foresight; the workforce-analytics engine aligns with federal workforce-stabilization priorities; and its continuous-learning design fulfills accreditation standards for performance-based public administration.

Strategic Pathways for U.S. Replication

1. Inter-County Modernization Cohorts

Neighboring rural counties can replicate Delaware's framework through shared data templates, dashboard architectures, and modernization workshops. Such cohorts lower implementation costs and create peer benchmarking for modernization progress.

2. State Technical Assistance and Incentives

State agencies should embed modernization readiness into grant scoring. Counties that operationalize analytics or transparency dashboards qualify for incremental performance funding—making modernization an earned investment rather than a compliance cost.

3. Institutional Learning Networks

Partnerships among universities, foundations, and regional planning councils can sustain modernization education. Delaware County's model provides the case study backbone for cross-county learning curricula that blend public-administration theory with applied analytics.

Cross-Border Application — Ontario and Beyond

Ontario's rural municipalities mirror Delaware's demographic aging, sparse connectivity, and data fragmentation. The Delaware framework's three-phase approach—Data Stabilization, Integration & Analytics, Learning Governance—offers a sequential pathway adaptable to Canadian administrative systems.

Through SozoRock's North American Rural Intelligence Program, U.S. counties and Ontario regional governments can exchange data-governance standards, co-develop analytics curricula, and jointly evaluate modernization outcomes. The initiative positions rural governance modernization as a continental resilience strategy rather than an isolated local reform.

Funding and Sustainability Mechanisms

Modernization durability depends on financial design that reinforces itself through measurable results. Delaware County's fiscal data show dependable but narrow revenue margins; sustainability therefore requires blended funding anchored in performance.

Recommended mechanisms

- **Performance-Linked Grants** — reward counties achieving verified modernization milestones.
- **Public-Private Partnerships** — enlist regional banks and analytics providers for infrastructure support.
- **Innovation Pilots** — secure foundation grants to test dashboard and interoperability prototypes.
- **Academic Collaborations** — leverage universities for data-science training and evaluation capacity.

Such diversification ensures modernization generates fiscal value through efficiency gains and improved public trust.

Institutional Scalability Model

Stage	County Readiness Level	Key Deliverables	Replication Mechanism
Stage 1 – Foundational Readiness	Counties maintaining verified datasets but minimal integration	Standardized templates, fiscal dashboards	State technical assistance
Stage 2 – Integrative Modernization	Counties with digital reporting systems	Workforce analytics tools, predictive budgeting models	Inter-county cohort training
Stage 3 – Adaptive Governance	Counties operating analytics teams	Continuous-learning loops, public transparency dashboards	National and binational exchange platforms

This modular design allows incremental adoption without overburdening small administrative units. Delaware County's disciplined implementation provides the first operational benchmark for this scalable pathway.

Figure 6

Scalability Matrix: County Readiness vs Replication

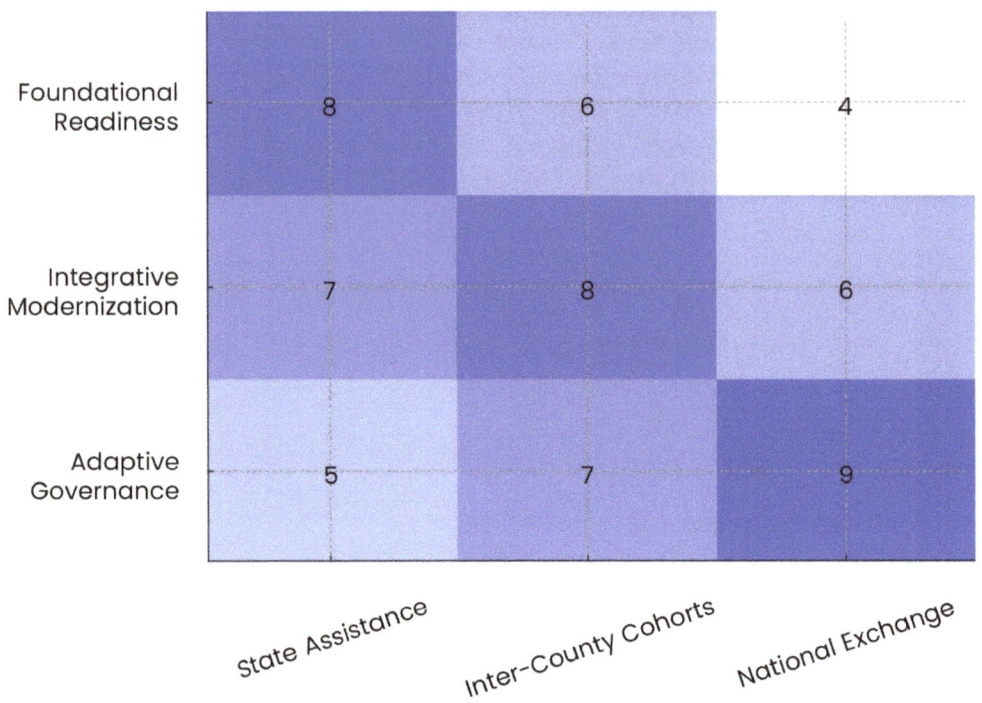

Source: SozoRock Foundation Systems Modernization Assessment (2025).

Counties at foundational readiness benefit most from state technical assistance, while adaptive jurisdictions excel through binational learning exchanges.

National Impact and Future Outlook

The Delaware County framework strengthens the nation's public-sector infrastructure through foresight and interoperability.

Short-term (1–2 years): measurable improvements in fiscal forecasting accuracy and staff retention.

Medium-term (3–5 years): institutionalization of learning governance practices across departments.

Long-term (5–10 years): creation of a rural-governance modernization ecosystem that informs federal policy and cross-border collaboration.

Replication Network Map:
New York and Ontario Knowledge Exchange

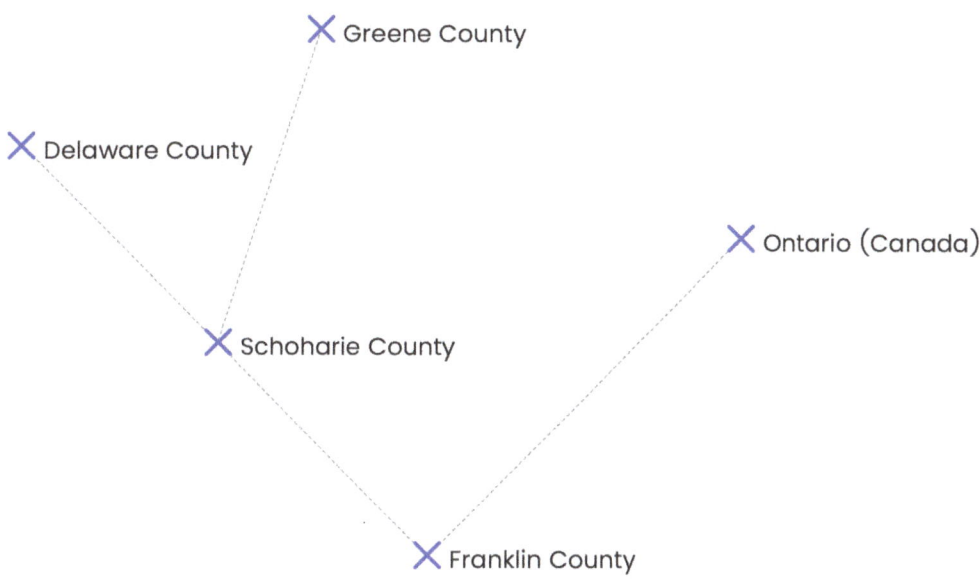

Source: SozoRock Foundation North American Rural Intelligence Program (2025).

Delaware County anchors the emerging cross-border modernization network, with knowledge transfer to peer New York counties and Ontario's rural systems.

Concluding Outlook

Modernization becomes durable when systems learn. Delaware County's progression from compliance to intelligence demonstrates that rural administrations can match the analytical sophistication of larger jurisdictions when transparency, data discipline, and foresight converge.

The Rethinking Rural Governance series positions SozoRock's framework as a cornerstone of modern rural administration—a structure through which counties across North America can evolve into adaptive institutions that continuously generate knowledge, anticipate risk, and reinforce the stability of national governance.

SozoRock®

Care. For Every Zip Code.

Emerging Models Strengthening Rural Systems

Rural communities advance when governance, access, and infrastructure reinforce one another. Two emerging models within The SozoRock Foundation's systems portfolio—CB-CAP and the Library Health Equity Hub (LHEH)—offer rural counties a practical, scalable way to improve how residents connect to essential services while reducing strain on local agencies. These models align with national priorities in public health modernization, digital equity, and rural workforce stabilization, making them suitable for counties across New York State, the broader United States, and communities in Northern Canada.

CB-CAP, the County-Based Community Access Platform, is a county-aligned structure that organizes health, social, and community resources into a clear, resident-facing access system. It helps counties simplify navigation, strengthen cross-sector coordination, and build a more predictable experience for residents seeking care, education, behavioral-health support, housing assistance, or digital tools. CB-CAP integrates easily with funding sources counties already use—public-health allocations, rural broadband programs, opioid settlement funds, and community-benefit resources from health systems—without requiring new physical infrastructure.

The Library Health Equity Hub extends the CB-CAP framework by positioning libraries as year-round access points for digital health, literacy, and community services. Libraries already serve as trusted public institutions, and the LHEH model enables them to support telehealth readiness, health education, digital navigation, program enrollment, and community engagement. The structure fits within existing library workflows and aligns with U.S. and Canadian privacy expectations, allowing rural regions in Ontario and British Columbia to adopt the model without major operational changes.

Both models contribute to the growing need for interdisciplinary training in rural systems. Universities—especially programs in occupational therapy, nursing, cybersecurity, health informatics, and public policy—can incorporate these frameworks into coursework, field placements, and applied research. The approach gives students and faculty a practical way to examine rural governance challenges while strengthening rural workforce pathways.

CB-CAP and the LHEH model help counties address chronic-disease burdens, geographic isolation, digital inequity, and workforce shortages through structures that can be scaled, funded, and adapted to local needs. These two models also establish a foundation for future work across rural systems, including Nursing Xchange, interdisciplinary professional pathways, and the upcoming health-systems assurance initiatives that focus on digital readiness and governance stability.

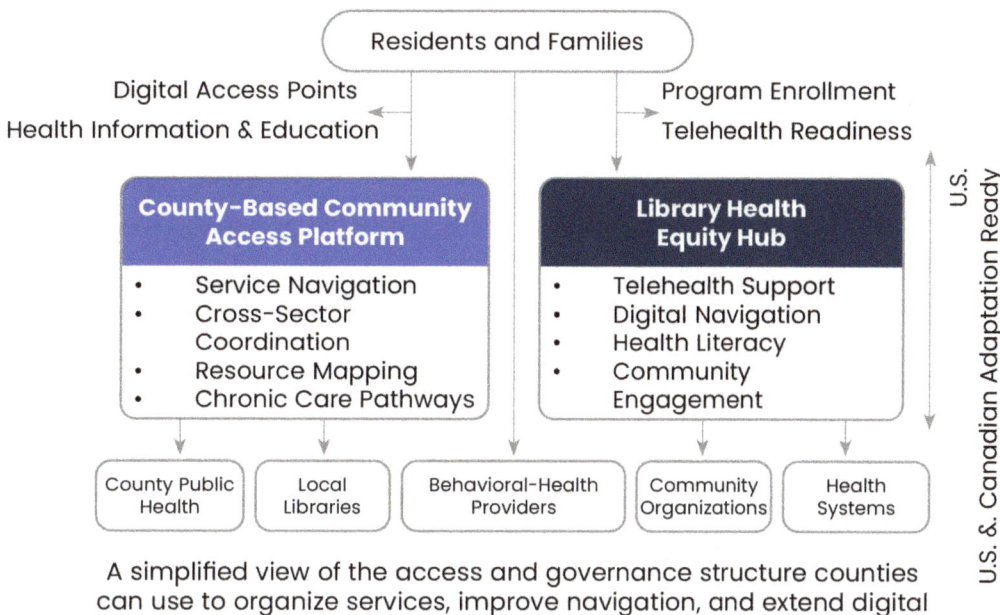

A simplified view of the access and governance structure counties can use to organize services, improve navigation, and extend digital health capacity

The diagram positions CB-CAP on the left side of the access layer to show its role as the county's organizing structure for service navigation, coordination, resource mapping, and chronic-care pathways. The upward arrows indicate how this structure strengthens digital access, health information, and resident-facing support, while the downward arrows show its reliance on county public health, libraries, behavioral-health providers, community organizations, and health systems. This expresses that CB-CAP does not replace county agencies—it organizes them into a clearer, more predictable access system for residents.

The Library Health Equity Hub appears on the right side of the access layer, parallel to CB-CAP, to reflect their shared function as complementary models. The diagram highlights the hub's role in telehealth support, digital navigation, health literacy, and community engagement—functions libraries can carry out within their current mandate when connected to CB-CAP. The upward arrows illustrate how the hub supports program enrollment and telehealth readiness for residents, while the downward arrows show its collaboration with libraries, behavioral-health providers, community groups, and health systems. This situates the hub at the intersection of digital literacy, public health, and community education.

Insight

High-trust institutions such as libraries accelerate digital adoption and strengthen chronic-care support when coordinated through a county-level access structure.

This structure can be adapted across rural U.S. counties and Northern Canadian regions with minimal change to existing workflows or governance requirements.

The workforce and professional pathways below sustain and operationalize the access models presented on the previous page.

Developing the Rural Workforce and Professional Pathways

Rural access systems depend on a workforce able to support digital navigation, chronic-care coordination, program enrollment, and community engagement. Two complementary structures—Nursing Xchange and Interdisciplinary Professional Pathways—expand the capability of local systems without requiring new capital infrastructure. They strengthen staffing predictability, broaden professional participation across disciplines, and reinforce the access models introduced on the previous page.

Nursing Xchange enables nurses to rotate across clinical sites, library hubs, behavioral-health locations, and community programs based on demand, training needs, and chronic-care priorities.

This gives counties a stable mechanism for addressing staffing gaps, preparing for seasonal or event-driven needs, and exposing nurses to digital tools and telehealth workflows. The model aligns with U.S. and Canadian practice expectations and can be supported through workforce grants, public-health allocations, and community-benefit funding.

Interdisciplinary Professional Pathways extend rural capacity by integrating occupational therapy, nursing, cybersecurity, informatics, public policy, and social-work learners into structured field experiences and capstones.

The framework provides universities with a practical way to align academic requirements with rural systems intelligence while giving counties additional support for digital navigation, chronic-care preparation, operational analysis, and community engagement. This helps early professionals contribute directly to local needs while strengthening the long-term talent pipeline.

These two models work alongside CB-CAP and the Library Health Equity Hub by supplying the staffing and interdisciplinary capability needed to sustain access, readiness, literacy, and program support throughout the year. They can be adapted across rural U.S. counties and northern Canadian regions with minimal changes to workflows or governance.

Nursing Xchange Workforce Mobility Model

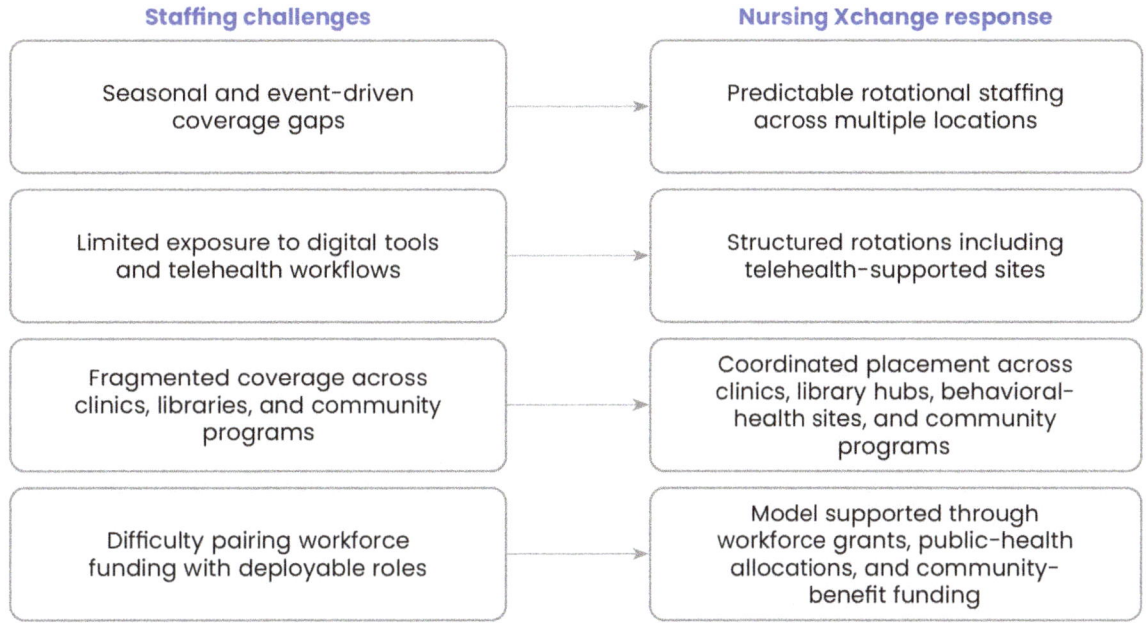

Nursing Xchange provides predictable rural staffing by rotating nurses across clinics, libraries, behavioral-health settings, and community programs while reinforcing chronic-care and telehealth readiness.

U.S. & Canadian adaptation ready

Interdisciplinary Professional Pathways

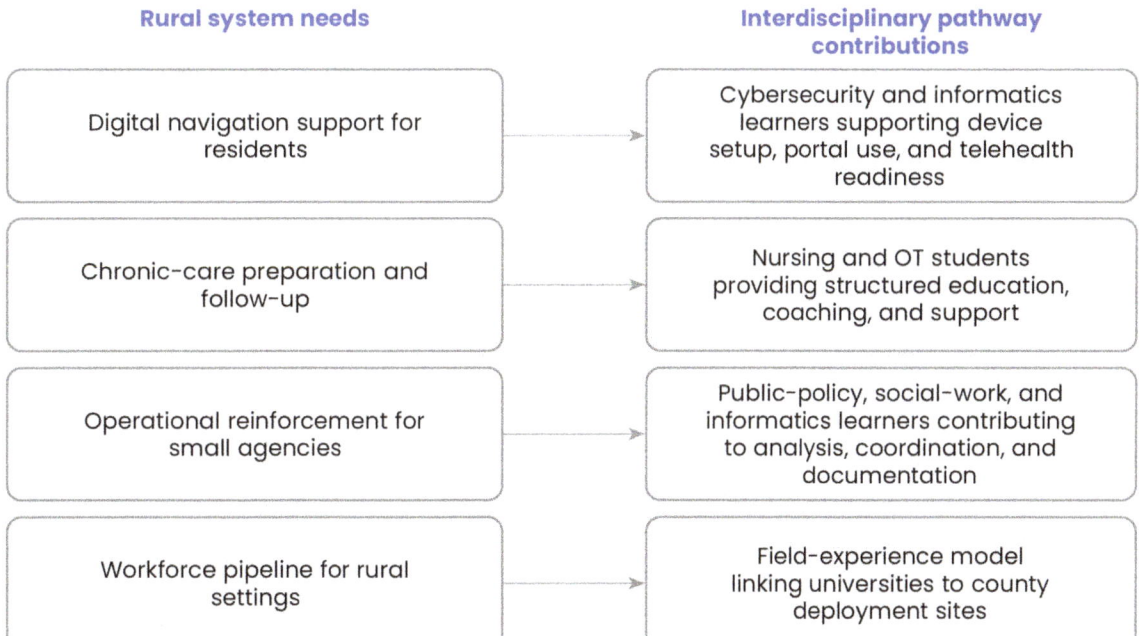

Interdisciplinary Professional Pathways align academic fields with rural system needs by translating learner capabilities into digital navigation, chronic-care support, and operational contributions across multiple community settings.

U.S. & Canadian adaptation ready

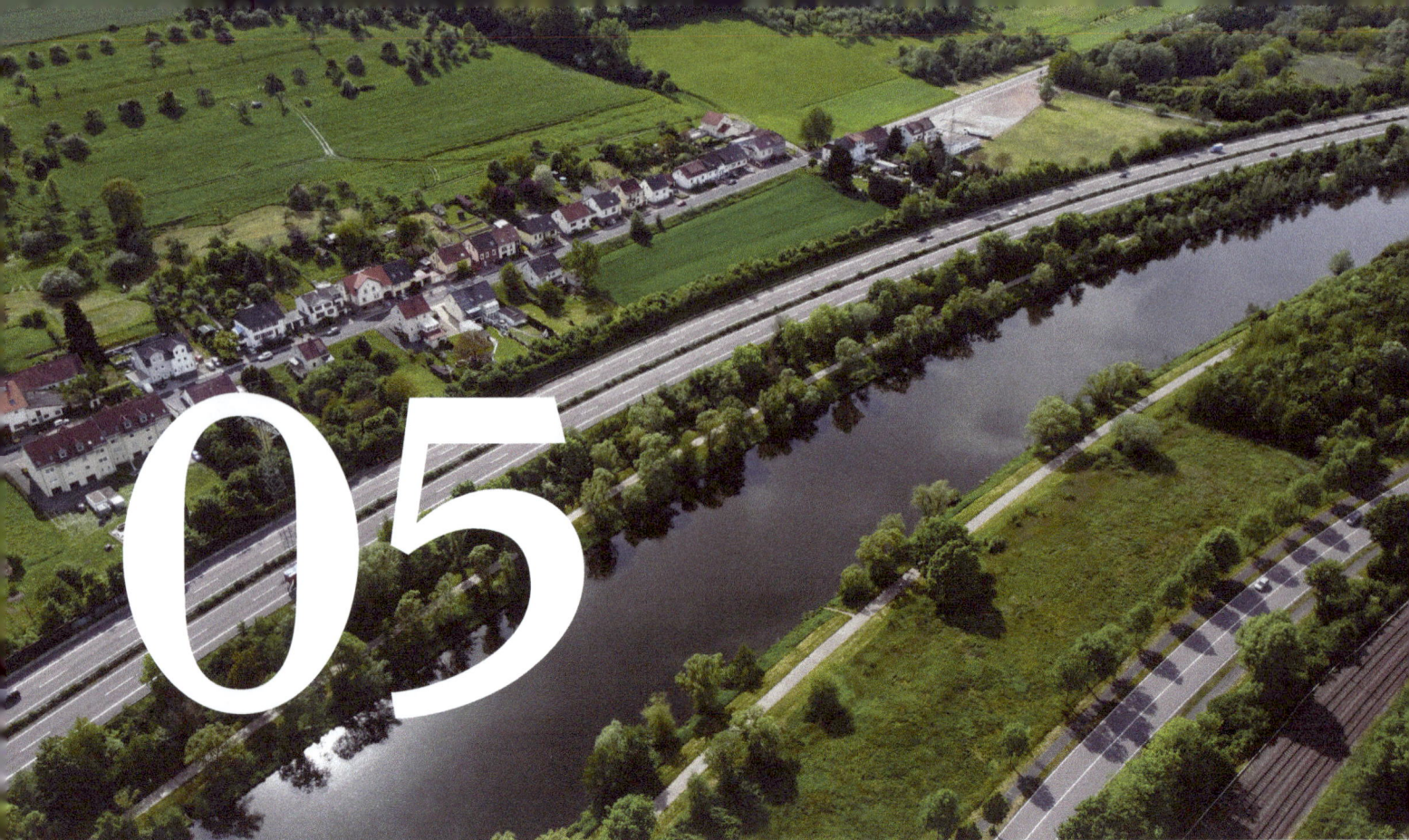

05

Appendices and Data References

Documentary Sources and Verification

All analytical insights in this report derive from verified public documents and administrative datasets published by Delaware County and affiliated agencies between 2022 and 2025. Each source was cross-validated through at least two independent records or board minutes to ensure accuracy, consistency, and traceability.

All analytical data in this report were verified against the following primary county and state documents.

Source Category	Primary Document / Record Set	Date / Period	Verification Purpose
Public Health Services Annual Report	Delaware County Public Health Services – 2024 Annual Report	FY 2024	Fiscal composition, expenditure pattern, program structure
Community Health Assessment / Improvement Plan	Delaware County CHA / CHIP 2022–2024	2022–2024	Demographic, chronic-disease, and social determinant baselines
Health Services Advisory Board Minutes	Verified sessions (January, March, June 2025)	2025	Governance oversight, workforce recruitment, and grant acceptance
County Fiscal and Budget Records	Finance Office statements and Article 6 grant documentation	2024–2025	Verification of state and federal aid ratios
Environmental Health Program Logs	Environmental Division reports	2024	Operational activity and inspection volumes
Emergency Preparedness Evaluations	County Preparedness After-Action Reviews	2024–2025	Coordination, simulation outcomes, and resource capacity mapping
Workforce and Infrastructure Grants	Public Health Infrastructure Grant documentation	2024–2025	Staffing and modernization alignment verification
State and Federal Frameworks	NYS Prevention Agenda 2025–2030; CDC Data Modernization Initiative	2023–2025	Comparative benchmark for modernization frameworks

Analytical Framework and Methodology

The Delaware County modernization analysis followed SozoRock's proprietary **Evidence → Interpretation → Lever** sequence used across all modernization diagnostics:

1. **Evidence Identification** — Verified all county records, fiscal tables, and board minutes to isolate measurable trends.
2. **Interpretation** — Analyzed patterns to determine governance constraints, operational strengths, and modernization potential.
3. **Lever Definition** — Mapped verified patterns to modernization levers — Fiscal Intelligence, Workforce Analytics, and Community Transparency — ensuring every insight derives from verifiable documentation rather than interpretive inference.

This process ensured that every insight presented in Sections 2–4 is derived directly from verifiable documentation rather than interpretive inference.

Framework Definitions and Terminology

Term	Operational Definition
Systems Intelligence	The institutional capability to transform operational data into predictive insight and continuous learning.
Modernization Lever	A measurable mechanism that produces efficiency, foresight, or resilience in administrative systems.
Continuous-Learning Governance	Governance practice where decisions generate new data that refine future policy design.
Data Integrity Cycle	The recurring validation and reconciliation process ensuring all administrative datasets remain accurate and interoperable.
Transparency Index	A public-reporting metric measuring the frequency and accessibility of validated governance dashboards.

Acknowledgments

The SozoRock Foundation recognizes the Delaware County Public Health Services leadership, administrative staff, and fiscal officers whose verified documentation provided the empirical base for this analysis.

Acknowledgment also extends to the Health Services Advisory Board for maintaining transparent, publicly accessible minutes and to New York State Department of Health for alignment with statewide modernization priorities.

All analyses, interpretations, and conclusions contained in this volume are the independent work of the SozoRock Foundation.

The Foundation acknowledges the professionalism of Delaware County officials whose transparency enabled this model for rural governance modernization.

Replication and Licensing Notice

This publication forms part of the **Rethinking Rural Governance** series, issued under **The SozoRock Foundation (New York)** imprint.

Materials may be cited or reproduced for educational and policy purposes with attribution. Derivative use or commercial adaptation requires written authorization.

Visuals, frameworks, and tables may be adapted for local-government training under a non-commercial license.

© 2025 The SozoRock Foundation – All Rights Reserved.

Printed in the United States of America.

Series Continuation Plan

The analytical model developed in Rethinking Rural Governance: Volume 1 — Delaware County, New York serves as the reference framework for future applications.

Subsequent volumes will adapt this methodology to additional New York counties and a cross-border Ontario pilot, strengthening the comparative evidence base for national and binational modernization.

Each release will align with The SozoRock Foundation's Modernization and Resilience Program, advancing equitable, data-driven governance and expanding the shared knowledge base that underpins rural systems intelligence.

Planned publication schedule subject to verification cycles and county collaboration agreements (2026–2027).

Each volume will replicate Delaware County's methodology to build a national and binational modernization knowledge base.

Citation and Contact Information

Publisher – The SozoRock Foundation (New York, USA)
Imprint – SozoRock Modernization and Resilience Program
Author – Oluwabiyi Adeyemo, MBA, DBA (Candidate) in Strategic Management
Series Title – Rethinking Rural Governance
Volume – Delaware County, New York — From Compliance to Systems Intelligence
ISBN – 979-8-9936477-1-5
Edition – First U.S. Edition (2025)

Preferred Citation:

Adeyemo, O. (2025). *Rethinking Rural Governance: Volume 1 – Delaware County, New York — From Compliance to Systems Intelligence.* The SozoRock Foundation, New York.

End Note

Modernization is not a single reform but a cumulative discipline. Delaware County's evolution—from procedural compliance to emerging systems intelligence—illustrates how data, governance, and learning converge to strengthen both local performance and national resilience.

Each insight in this volume stands as evidence that when governance learns, communities thrive.

Rural Equity Blueprint Series

SozoRock®
Care. For Every Zip Code.

Advancing rural health equity through data, workforce renewal, and governance modernization

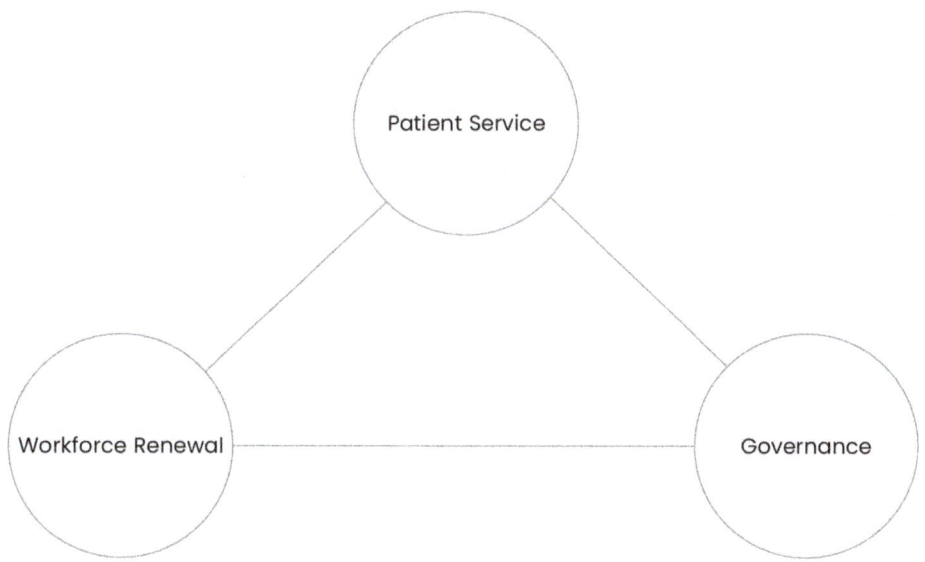

The Rural Equity Blueprint Series (REBS) anchors The SozoRock Foundation's U.S. modernization program on equitable access and measurable outcomes across medically underserved counties.

Volume 1 — Access Day:
Building a Framework for Rural Health Equity in New York State defines a triad model — Patient Service · Workforce Renewal · Governance — that transforms equity intent into operational design.

Each edition applies verified data and systems-intelligence methods to align community health needs with fiscal and workforce strategies. The series supports state and federal grant alignment, Medicaid 1115 waiver pilots, and cross-county modernization plans that advance community resilience.

REBS contributes an empirical foundation for evidence-driven rural-governance reform and complements the modernization frameworks advanced in Rethinking Rural Governance (Vol. 1).

JANUARY 2026 FEATURE
A SozoRock Systems Spotlight

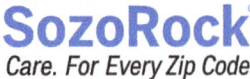

HEALTH SYSTEMS ASSURANCE (HSA)
Building digital trust across modern health infrastructure

Applied Foundation

The assurance pathway is designed and led by Oluwabiyi Adeyemo, who directs the graduate-level cybersecurity capstone delivered in collaboration with Capella University's Cybersecurity Graduate Faculty. The Fall 2025 instructional phase introduces five master's-degree candidates—located across Eastern, Central, and Mountain time zones—to structured assurance tasks inside SozoRock's secured cloud environment, where Adeyemo provides direct leadership, technical guidance, and evaluation.

The Spring 2026 phase advances the work into live practical implementation, with students validating controls and documenting assurance evidence under Adeyemo's direction. The model strengthens national readiness by showing how education, systems intelligence, and governance discipline can operate in a unified assurance environment.

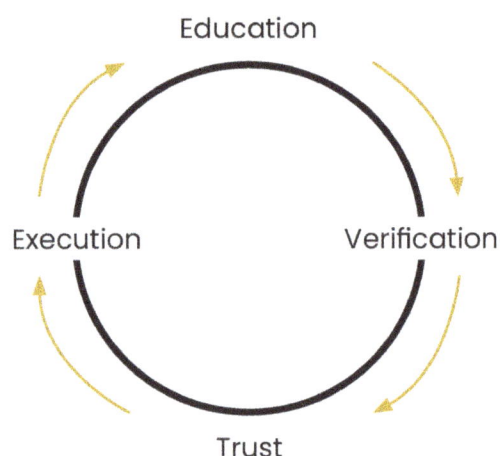

Insight

Insights from this instructional and implementation model inform the assurance framework authored in *Digital Assurance (2026)*, where verification, systems intelligence, and governance discipline are treated as core elements of national health-system resilience. The work demonstrates how a structured assurance pathway—rooted in education, supervised practice, and validated controls—can strengthen public-interest infrastructure across U.S. and allied health environments.

Authored by
Oluwabiyi Adeyemo, MBA
Director of Strategic Initiatives — The SozoRock Foundation

© 2025 The SozoRock Foundation
HIPAA • SOC 2 • NIST 800-53 • PHIPA
Conducted in academic collaboration with Capella University Cybersecurity Graduate Faculty (Fall 2025 instructional phase; Spring 2026 practical phase)

www.ingramcontent.com/pod-product-compliance
Lightning Source LLC
Chambersburg PA
CBHW040005040426
42337CB00033B/5234